Franz Guenter Leicht

Personal experience with the Kundalini energy and spiritual backgrounds

franzguenter-leicht.info

Publisher: **Leicht Franz Guenter**, 52 pages, b/w, 1 figure

To acquire e.g. via **www.lulu.com or www.amazon.de**

Cover design: Franz Guenter Leicht

Press: Lulu Press, Inc.
           3101 Hillsborough Street
           Raleigh, NC 27607
           United States

ISBN: 978-1-326-56423-0

1. Edition.

Content.

Introduction.

We live in a time in which an energetic influence can be observed, which is probably as strong as never before. To be mentioned are electromagnetic pollution; the vibrational field of the collective; energy of the Photon Belt, in which our solar system penetrates more and more; subtle and spiritual energies which surround us and energy changes within our aura system. *In terms of our spiritual development, not all energies are conducive.*

If we observe our life, sometimes it seems as if the energy is not even kept balanced and that instead, those energies gain the upper hand, which oppose our spiritual development. Nevertheless, I think that this principle does not have to be that way. We have the choice to come in resonance with the one or the other kind of energy, as we turn our attention to the corresponding energy. This of course requires a constant vigilance.

A not to be underestimated factor in influencing energy is the expansion of the aura of man. The aura of the man may be more or less extended. If the aura is barely expanded, it can hardly protect us from the low-energy and self-destructive energies that surround us. Because then, these energies can permeate our energy-body system easier or can adhere to it (possession ?). We are then constantly influenced by these energies and must constantly go against them. This can be noticed that we feel hardly a change with our positive thoughts, with our prayers and affirmations, although a change is of course there.

It is different if we have a strong extended aura. Such an aura shields us from the low-energy and self-defeating thoughts of people as well as from other low-energy vibrations. This can be noticed that we can achieve our goals faster and easier and that we can go through life much easier. With a strong extended aura other effects are associated. In a highly extended aura the energy centers, the so-called chakras, are developed as optimal antennas to be receptive for higher dimensional energies, which makes possible the connection to the cosmic consciousness. If our aura is extended optimally (100%), which corresponds to a range of several hundred meters, one kilometer or more, then subtle higher dimensional energies can flow freely through our aura system. Then our energy body system is as a superconductor and allows us to bring energy from the subtle level to the material level with ease. People with a 100% strength developed Aura presumably can materialize things or accomplish things that could be classified as a miracle: to be immune to deadly poisons, walk on water, turning water into wine and so on.

The question now is how we can bring our aura for expanding. Here there are again many possibilities, for example, if we are open to everything. If we are open to everything, we stretch out quasi our sensor unlimited. Thus, the Aura has a tendency to expand. Moreover, if we release of tensions or other things that virtually put us in bondage and that do not let us live in the flow stream of life, we allow the energy to flow into our Aura system. By this the aura has also a tendency to expand. We can imagine that we emit energy far away into the world, so that we are even the far radiant aura.

Certainly the energies which are emitted from the cosmos (ever-increasing radiation by the penetration of our solar system into the Photon Belt, other cosmic events) contribute as well to the fact that we will more and more be filled with energy. On the other hand, the majority of people seems increasingly to fall into anxiety, fear and struggle, which, inter alia, is evoked outright by dark forces. In this way the two forces seem more or less balance each other, so that things cannot change fundamentally. We can consciously escape the dark influence by following our internal plan/ our intuition as a neutral observer which is without fear, full of confidence and full of courage.

Regarding the expansion of the aura the Kundalini energy of man plays an important role. It must be said that this energy is in every human being. It is a subtle energy that quasi has rested or slept for most people in the past and thereby has been entirely unnoticeable. In a time of increased exposure of energy and the self-development this energy will be awoken in man in a strengthened way: in the one more in the other less.

So the Kundalini will be active on the one hand or can "lie dormant" as potential energy in us on the other hand. If the Kundalini-energy lies dormant, it has the form of a ball lightning. In the form of a ball lightning it is directed at nothing, i.e. it causes no damage or doesn't influence anything. So in this case we do not notice anything of it. But once parts thereof are peeled off from the ball gradually, more and more Kundalini energy starts to flow. These peeled parts of the Kundalini energy ensure that they gradually dissolve the energy blockades of the aura system. There are visualization and other exercises which cause this peeling (see the Kundalini Manual "Kundalini and the Chakras", Genevieve Lewis Paulson). <u>Keywords:</u> Kundalini-triggering which can be brought about spontaneously or deliberately. One can say that the aura cannot regress under the influence of the Kundalini energy. The Kundalini stabilizes the aura system. The more Kundalini energy flows, the further the aura is extended and developed. For example, I once read that in Jesus the Kundalini is said to be up to 80% in flux. Because the aura of Jesus was so strongly developed, he presumably could work miracles, which have been reported.

As to whether the aura can also be extended without Kundalini energy, I got following thoughts. Without Kundalini energy perhaps we would have to live in a secluded place or even in a place of high force (place of power), have constantly to meditate and/or constantly to call high forces. This is practically hardly possible in a busy world. Therefore it stands to reason that in a busy society we have really to need the Kundalini energy to stabilize the aura, whereby we are able at any time to tackle with ease against the destructive forces, which surround us, or even to raise above these forces without that we struggle.

In terms of our spiritual development, for example, the influence of all possible artificial radiations (electromagnetic pollution), the high deficiency of nutrients and trace elements in our food, the various toxins to that we are exposed, an executed way of life against the biorhythm and the like more seem not to be negligible. This does not mean that the just explained is actually harmful to us, but that this might bind our mind to the matter. Without these things our mind would probably be much free. At least these things can never contribute to let unfold our aura or let work the inner processes in our energy body system without resistance. As long as our energy body system suffers blockades, it lacks of supply of our organs with vital energy, what we have to balance on the material plane in any form. With a fully developed aura, our energy body system is like a superconductor, which can let flow the subtle and higher dimensional energies into our energy body system without resistance, which frees us largely from terrestrial dependencies. In my view without Kundalini energy it would be hardly possible, particularly in the Western world, to bring our Aura system fully to unfold or to extend. Of course, the existence of Kundalini speaks for itself.

Well it should be noted that the Kundalini energy is a very powerful energy. If our energy body system is not prepared for this energy it can bring serious crises with itself. Once excessive Kundalini triggering is done, then the energy body system can be so strong muddled up that for a certain time we stand between life and death, and we have no influence on the course. Here, a mental control is practically hardly possible. **Therefore, it is advisable to learn to feel when we have to work really with this energy!!!**

We just live in a time in which the inner desire of people for spiritual development increases more and more. Once the aura system of people is prepared in relation to the Kundalini energy and there is also a strong inner urge for spiritual development, then the Kundalini energy will be noticeable as if by magic. For me it started about 20 years ago as follows. At that time I began to meditate a lot. One day, half asleep, I heard a message that internal forces would deploy in me. Initially it was not at all clear for me, how this would be done. A few days later during meditations I repeatedly perceived how energy hissed through my body, as if a lightning bolt hissed through my body. At first I thought that this is a hypersensitivity, if someone in the house - at that

12

time I lived in a large tenement - switched on the light (by the light switch). Of course I could not verify this.

At that time I was already looking for various topics that I wanted to deal, such as Channeling, Kundalini, Esoteric and other things. I had about 3 or 4 topics. For this purpose I wrote the corresponding terms in a star shape on a piece of paper and I consulted an oracle (pendulum). The pendulum was directed to the term "Kundalini". I knew there was a handbook to this energy. So, I bought it to read. Among other things, these flashes of light in the body were described there as a symptom of Kundalini-triggering which can occur spontaneously or, for example, may be initiated by the Holy Spirit. Anyone who has problems with the term "Holy Spirit", whom should be said that such trigger may be initiated by a higher consciousness Instance from us. So, it isn't really important which name we give this instance.

For whom is this working-out intended?

If you have to deal with symptoms that hardly anyone understands, not even the doctors. If in your aura system something happens that no one can really empathize. If the Kundalini energy is misdirected in you and you are now and then confronted with symptoms for which you can find no common explanation. If you have no one with whom you can talk about the Kundalini energy. Then this working-out could be a little help. Now, it helps already enormously, if you know what other people have experienced in connection with this energy. *Moreover, you should know that it will mostly come to a good end. This energy assists you enormously on your spiritual path.* The Kundalini is a guarantee that you do not stand still and that you can always continue to go ahead spiritually, unless that you willfully put an end to your life.

I had hesitated long time to publish this document, because I thought that there is to read enough on the subject "Kundalini energy". But perhaps this document is important, interesting and also helpful precisely **for those people, in which the Kundalini energy has taken a misguided path similar to mine**. Also, I suspect that this is not the case with a few people. We're living in a time of spiritual liberation, where the Kundalini energy is gaining in importance more and more.

Because I myself have collected experience over 20 years with the Kundalini energy, I think that this working-out can make guts for all those who are faced with symptoms that they cannot explain. Of course not all non-diagnosable symptoms (according to conventional medicine) are traceable to the Kundalini energy. For example, there are also so-called Light Body symptoms. But I think that the Kundalini does not have insignificant influence to such symptoms.

Perhaps it's not so important to know what exactly the causes are. Often, it is sufficient to know that these symptoms are part of an overall purification process that wants to lead us more and more to our true divinity. ***Because energy will be incorporated in our energy body system in this process, our body system itself must be adapted and adjusted to these changes.*** And, depending on how strong the respective energy flows are, that adaption can cause different difficulties for the body system which may manifest itself by certain symptoms of body and/or of state of mind.

Note: If you experience symptoms at you, for those there is no medical explanation, then it does not necessarily mean that the Kundalini energy is awakened in you. Because there are also so-called Light Body symptoms that are not medically explicable. But if the Kundalini energy is awakened in you, it may well appear symptoms, which are not diagnosable by the conventional medicine. Because, if the Kundalini energy awakens in you, it has the tendency to dissolve all energy blockades. And, depending on the activity of the Kundalini energy, in certain circumstances this dissolution can be painful or can make you pretty messed up.

Nevertheless, if the Kundalini energy is involved in a development process, we should always be aware of the fact that this can be a great blessing for us, maybe with a few exceptions. To understand this better, let us do the following considerations.

The path between heaven and hell or why we have the feeling to <u>tread water.</u>

1. We are surrounded by all kinds of energies. One could say that we are in an energy water, which contains all possible frequencies, from very low to infinitely high.
2. At the low frequencies we speak for simplicity of low, dark energies that do us no good (blockades, dense energies that impose us limits). At the high frequencies we talk about clear, harmonious energies that are good for us and that open the borders.
3. We are somewhere between the two types of energies that affect us simultaneously. Seen Illustrates we are a mixed water, which results from the mixing of cold and hot water.
4. The hot water symbolizes the high, bright energy. The cold water symbolizes the low, "dark" energy.
5. The question is: **"How can we let carry us from the high bright energy and can let detach ourselves from the low "dark" energy?"**
6. The simple answer is: **"By directing my attention to freedom, harmony, joy and love!!!"**

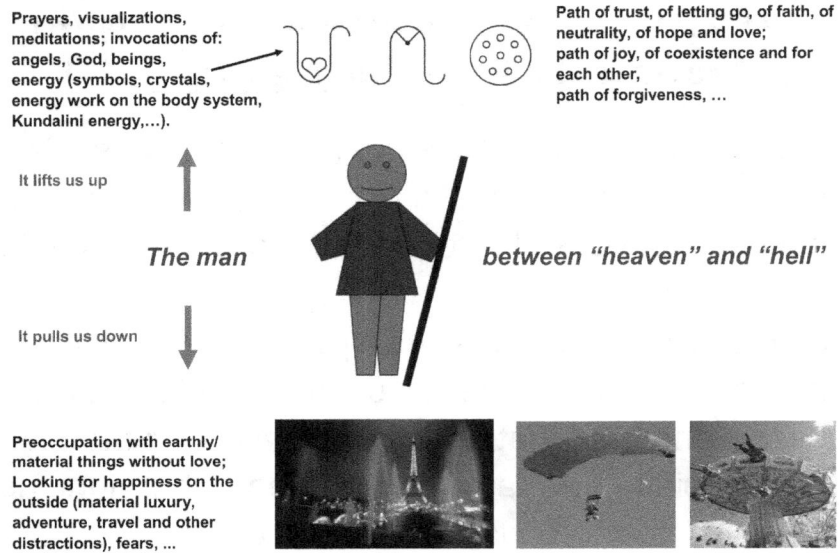

Prayers, visualizations, meditations; invocations of: angels, God, beings, energy (symbols, crystals, energy work on the body system, Kundalini energy,...).

Path of trust, of letting go, of faith, of neutrality, of hope and love; path of joy, of coexistence and for each other, path of forgiveness, ...

It lifts us up

The man

between "heaven" and "hell"

It pulls us down

Preoccupation with earthly/ material things without love; Looking for happiness on the outside (material luxury, adventure, travel and other distractions), fears, ...

For this purpose, here the following clear proportionalities: If I reject something, I direct my attention to what I don't want to have. So I build a resonance with the corresponding energies. By that, I bind myself to this thing/energy (which I don't want) and create the tendency to attract it formally. So, rejection is not the right way. It is better to accept everything, because it already surrounds me energetically. If I recollect on my inner impulses and on my true nature at the same time, I come into resonance with the clear, harmonious part of me or of the universe. In this case, it lifts me energetically upwards as if by magic. The result is that I allow the higher, clear energy to dissolve blockades and to harmonize parts of my body system. If a progressive harmonization of my energy body-system takes place, a healing process can be set in motion.

Conclusion: By reflecting on ourselves and on the embassies in us, as well by listening to the inner impulses, an improvement of our lives takes place at all possible levels.

Here very briefly the various things that are helping us in this way:

- Trust, forgiveness, love
- To enjoy your life
- To pamper body and soul
- To muster courage to live your life and not to live the other's life
- Prayers / affirmations / mantras
- Visualizations
- Meditations and breathing exercises
- Energy work on the body, working with symbols (light crystals)
- Kundalini
- …

At the very moment in which I get into mischief, in fear, anger or doubt I can make me aware that I have a choice of attention to absolve me energetically from the low-energy vibrations. I can do it by the prayer, for example to say positive things (affirmations, mantras) or by imagining in spirit, how it feels, to live in fortune, in wealth and prosperity.

Now we know the saying that a picture says more than thousand words. It is similar with the use of prayers, affirmations and visualizations. If I can take pictures of desired goals and connect them with a positive feeling in the mind, then I can do more than only by the application of thousand prayers, affirmations or mantras. If I succeed to make this visualization in deep meditation while my mood is extremely good, then the desire can realize the objectives abruptly. For this one must come into a vibrational state, in which the brain emits waves between 4 and 8 Hz (theta waves) or waves below 5 Hz (delta waves).

If it is not possible for us to come into such a deep state, we are trying to settle down, to make these visualizations for maybe at least 7 minutes. This we can do at best before we are going to bed and immediately after waking up.

In some ways, desires and visualizations are a kind of plea or request. If we have a request which is expressed out from a lack feeling, we can assume that the thoughts and feelings that are hidden behind them, have a much stronger force that usually preclude our request. Then we can assume that it's hardly possible to achieve our goals according to our Please. Therefore it's often said to express our petition in a state of relaxation, happiness and confidence. The request should be expressed as if everything already happened or at least is potentially available. Accordingly, a request can be applied only then successfully, if it is really a prayer of thanks. In other words, the greater the feeling you have that this or that has already been done, and the more this feeling can be emitted in gratitude and in joy, the easier it is to manifest this or that.

It should be said that there is nothing we have not already created in the spirit. Everything is potentially available. If we perceive this or that, it therefore has to do on what we draw our attention with all our conscious and unconscious thoughts, feelings and ideas. Since much is unconscious, our conscious mind has the feeling as if we were exposed to our fate. So, we are like unconscious creators. Others would say that we are caught in the matrix.

Of course, the request is not limited to material things. It can also be expanded to things like the connectivity with our true selves and the awareness of our divinity. Here it would be to say that we have the following advantages in the awareness of our divinity. By this awareness we know our true destiny, do really know what goals are worthwhile for us and we can achieve these objectives without much meditation exercises, so with ease. In addition, we are in this state no longer unconscious creators but conscious creators. The others would say that we are then dropped out of the matrix.

To get into the state of awareness of our divinity, which is likely to be the end goal of our soul, there are several possibilities. As I said, we can express our request as this was already done, what is really indeed so. Because in reality there is no energetic and no communicative separation. This separation seems to be only in a dream. So, this prayer of thanks is like a springboard to wake up. In a way the prayer of thanks allows us to be raised up energetically, because we let the higher and clear energies flow into our energy body system, which raises up also the collective energy. Metaphorically viewed our combined sewer warms up.

Now the prayer of thanks is one of several ways of increasing energy. Another possibility is the use of symbols, behind which positive energies are hidden. The so-called light crystals are symbols behind which angel beings and deities hide. Depending on the task these beings contribute in themselves energies of love, of fullness, of patience, of healing, of purification, of power etc. By involving ourselves with these crystals, for example, through visualization or by drawing (mentally or with hand) or by inhalation, we call over (invoke) these beings (= energy) to act in us or through us.

If we invoke them in this way, then they help us immediately with their energies according to their task areas. To my knowledge there is an agreement with our core/ with our soul that we get the corresponding aid or energy or messages if we use these crystals (symbols). The whole world of light is available to us, that we may call over it and that we shape the life on earth in loving and luminous way with it. In this way we bring down the heaven to the earth. It is perfectly legitimate to invite natural forces or spiritual powers, so that they interact with us (we with them, and they with us). **GOD'S idea of power resides precisely in the sharing of objectives with all its parts, which we are part of him.**

Well, after quantum physics principle every little part contains the whole. By applying this principle to our reality, we can say that we are not only part of God but also God. The part of God (all of us) is God (the whole). And so we can say, if we call any sorts of energies that we ultimately access aspects which are not really foreign but part of us.

When using light crystals, which indeed is only an access to a part of our overall aspect, we can be sure that the result of our efforts is not to the detriment of the whole. Let us remember here that the strength and power by using the crystals of light is greater than the strength and power by using symbols for selfish purposes (black magic). So why not prefer light crystals instead other symbols?

So we have a variety of ways we can transform our lives for good. It is sufficient to apply such means that we can easily do currently, or which do us offer precisely. Everything can be tried.

The Subtle.

Now, in case that statements are made about the Subtle, this does not mean that we are dealing with speculation, which would be completely unfounded. On the contrary, the knowledge of physics, according to which the universe is only about 4% of visible matter, confirm the existence of the Subtle. So the physics comes to the conclusion that the universe consists not only of visible matter but also of dark matter and of dark energy. From a physical standpoint, the term "dark" means, that we have to do with things that are not visible or directly observable with physical measurements. Dark matter and dark energy therefore are understood as the unseen or the invisible, which outweighs with its share of 94% by far the visible matter.

The knowledge of physics is largely limited to 4%, will mean that the remaining 96% are poorly understood. However, it is not so, that there is absolutely no evidence or information, which are attributable to this great rest area. On the contrary, here the Spiritual sciences provide a lot of information.

For example we know the term aura. Some people can see the aura or perceive it in another way. This suggests that the aura system is attributed to the area of the dark energy and/or dark matter. Incidentally, the aura system now is relatively well known. Mention should be made the book "The Subtle Body" by Cyndi Dale, which, to my knowledge, delivers the most thoroughly worked out summary of the subtle energy body of man. In conjunction with the aura system, there are concepts like Kundalini energy, chakras, meridians and subtle energy body. In my view, in the above mentioned book the closer links (connection) between the subtle energy body system and the body organs are very well described. Also, there are a lot of other literature on this links (connections) that we find if we look for the corresponding terms.

If there are disturbances in the subtle area, to the physical and mental level phenomena (symptoms) are noticeable, which often no longer fit in the diagnosis of classical medicine. Finally, personal testimonies have shown with such phenomena that the classical medicine or the classic psychotherapy cannot always find plausible explanations without the involvement of the Subtle. Personally, since more than 20 years I perceive subtle operations on my own energy body system and I'm faced with corresponding phenomena on the physical realm. Since that time I was also in exchange with several people who reported about phenomena, for that classical medicine or the classic psychotherapy had no plausible answers or solutions. **These testimonies have led me to publish this document.** So in this working-out I would like to present some relationships between the Subtle and the coarse visible matter.

Again: If the visible matter is only a small part of the wholeness it is very obvious to say that the subtle range influences the matter. **All the more, classical medicine and classical psychotherapy would be well advised to consider the subtle for the diagnostics.**

We live in an age in which such phenomena and symptoms accumulate, for which classical medicine and classic psychotherapy in my view has no adequate solutions. It is often so that such phenomena are coming out of the blue and go again, without a specific injury or inflammation can be observed on the body. Who is confronted with such phenomena, may conceivably fall into fear or panic, if he doesn't know the backgrounds (underlying cause). But, if he would have at least a little insight on the underlying causes, he would rather stay calm and would be rather able to take the right measures. Therefore, this document is intended to point out possible backgrounds and to take away the fear to people. Fear is not always a good counselor.

Personal experiences with the Kundalini energy.

Well, if the Kundalini energy is awakened in you, whether you know it or not, symptoms may occur out of the blue, without that you can fix a cause of it. I want to report from my own experience with the Kundalini energy, so you have an idea about what can happen.

It all started as I perceived a flash of light in the body from time to time in meditation or in a relaxed state. Mostly it was just a short light-like hiss of energy through my body, out of the blue. After I had triggered Kundalini for the first time by means of a visualization exercise I perceived something in the tailbone area that felt as if I had laid an egg. This egg felt viscous. Then this liquid divided. One part of it then wandered through my body, as if this part was led systematically. A little later I noticed that something pricked on the body surface for a short time. It picked each time at a different location. Then it started up to turn. I suspected that one chakra after another chakra was activated, of which there should be thousands. I noticed that I could rotate these chakras counter-clockwise or clockwise, as I wanted. I also could stop this turning. Probably I had overdone it with the conscious turning, because the next day it was me dizzy all day long.

Then I found that I could smell something that was previously not possible for me. I could smell very intensively people and plants. Women usually smelled sweetly and children even sweeter. I have also met people who smelled unpleasant. I suspected that people with the unpleasant odor were somehow sick. Likewise, my sense of taste was sharpened. Water tasted sweet. Well, this exceptional taste and smell, I lost after a few months.

The next observation was that something became detached slightly from my body, and that this detachment made a twist motion. It was as if a bunch of hair thin aura layers had been tied around my whole body whole the time like twisted wires. Then I suspected that these thin aura layers were gradually unfolded by the influence of the Kundalini energy. Over time, these layers always felt thicker and more viscous until solid. I tried to understand what it has to do with the development of auric layers. So I considered a model, as follows.

The aura of a man who is fully developed will have an expansion of more than one kilometer. This means that the aura extends over this enormous scope as an energetic structure. Now, the aura itself is composed of many auric layers which are nested one in the other, in which the higher energetic aura layers penetrate and outshine the energetically lower auric layers. For me, it was at first so that my aura had only a slight expansion, perhaps up to a maximum of a few meters. Maybe even less than one meter. The precise value isn't really relevant. **It is crucial that a weak expanded aura must be extremely compressed (forced together) compared to what it may have at the maximum expansion.** It is as if these individual layers are spirally twisted (tortuous) very close to the body. Based on my observation, it seemed as if the individual layers were/are simultaneously pressed, tied and glued; with all variations thereof. So, to let expand this compacted aura, layer by layer must be unfolded and unpeeled gradually. This is exactly what the Kundalini energy seems to do as if by magic, by flowing through more and more energy channels.

About 20 years ago in a session with a medium through which I could ask my guardian angel, I was told that my aura would unfold. Metaphorically speaking, a hard nut, similar to an almond nut shell, has to be cracked until the aura can expand. In my view this metaphor fits very well into the picture of a highly compacted aura. A compacted aura would be like an energetic armor that we had built around us. Had we built it around us for protection? If we built this for reasons of protection, then surely because of a misunderstanding. We wanted possibly to differentiate from others or to hide ourselves away? The downside is that by this energetic armor we had disconnected us at the same time from the surrounding cosmic energies and thus we lost the connection to our higher self.

The aura as a whole I could never perceive. I suspect that what is dense and virtually (still) immobile, is not perceptible with the inner sense. Probably only what is peeled layer by layer, and thus comes in dynamics, is perceptible (with the inner sense). The energy pathways of those layers which are dense, are energetically not flow-capable. Thus, such layers are full of energy blockades which can be gradually dissolved by the pulsing Kundalini energy, after it was once set free. This resolution of blockades can be perceived indirectly through the change in the aura and the associated symptoms (concomitants of the Kundalini process).

Concomitants of my Kundalini process were as follows: Two or three times a year I had severe stomach upset in connection with a headache for about 3-4 days. During this short time, I was almost all the time in bed. Or it came to pain which was caused by previous injuries which were themselves not yet healed completely. This pain stopped after a short time. For this it should be mentioned an injury to the meniscus which I had suffered several years ago while playing soccer. The pain of this meniscus came once again back for a few days, without overloading my knee. Furthermore, once I had about 2-3 weeks chest pain, as if I had been pierced by several daggers. This pain came out of the blue (without injury), but disappeared as if by magic. It was as if an event from a past life was going to come to light again, and then have to be reconciled once and for all. Or I even got relatively severe pain in the gastrointestinal region, which also came out of the blue, but to disappear after a few days. Here's to say that for a long time I had problems in the gastrointestinal area presumably in conjunction with an intestinal fungus.

During my Kundalini process I found more side effects (concomitants), which probably stood in connection with the influence of the Kundalini energy, as follows: From time to time I felt pretty tired and worn. From time to time energy hissed again flashed through my body. Sometimes I suddenly remembered to certain situations that I had experienced in this life. Once, I even reminded me of a previous birth, which proceeded in my mind's eye by an animated film which gave me to understand that there was an imminent birth. Although I am a man, I could also feel in my body, as if I were pregnant. I could feel the rapid movements of the child. Then I could see from the animated film that the birth was imminent. I quickly realized that it should be to my own birth. After a short break, I heard a voice, which probably came from my former father who appeared to me very jealous. I could not see anything. I can't remember anymore, what he said exactly, but I could feel that his hatred rendered on me. The feeling of not being wanted imprinted in the form of a certain pain in my stomach region. This type of pain came into this life, whenever I had the feeling of having done something wrong or not being loved.

If I was a bit relaxed, I always could feel the various changes to my aura system in conjunction with the Kundalini energy and I tended to pay great attention to this change. For a while it was so that this kept me literally engross, simply because it is always fascinating what was going on in my body. Then other things were less important, although they would certainly have been also important. For example, this "sympathizing with it" let me often not fall asleep, even though I felt tired. Here, then I would recommend not to let too much be monopolized by the influence of the Kundalini energy.

If I make a recap of all these 21 years, I can well say that the Kundalini process went relatively harmless comparatively to what I had heard from other people. In what way and to what intensity such concomitants make noticeable, it can vary greatly from person to person. Therefore caution is always on offer in case that you are working with the Kundalini energy. The better the aura system is prepared for the Kundalini process, the less problems are there in connection with the Kundalini energy.

In order to be well prepared for this process, the regular energy working on our own energy body system can be very useful. There are many ways to can do this. In the Chakra Handbook of Sharamon, Shalia & Baginski and Bodo J. you will find a very good compilation. Of course, not all of the disciplines described therein should be made. **Everyone should pick out of these many ways exactly what suits him best.** Rather take fewer things in attack, but do they well, than to do many things and make them bad. Here it is, in fact, to learn sensing what keeps us moving forward on this issue. Then, someday will come the impulse to deal directly with the Kundalini energy. Please, this also to learn to feel!!! **I think, the Kundalini is one of the greatest gift we have got.**

Interpretation of the pain, which is emerging again out of the blue.

If symptoms occur out of the blue, this could mean that the corresponding internal settings or beliefs (unpurified past) are now ready to be transferred into the light, to speak, to be rethought, so that we gradually come into a state of mind that corresponds to God's nature. It is to say, that God's nature is also our all nature.

In the course of this harmonization the unpurified past will be purified as if by magic, in which the pain of old injuries rise briefly again in weakened form and without real damage, so that it can be lighted from new. Only then, if in this new lighting we can bring the former wrong thinking and feeling back in the right light, we can let go of it. Then the old disharmonious seeming information will be converted (transformed) into a new harmonious seeming information what brings us in a (more) relaxed mindset and brings the cells of our body in the growth state or may hold them in this state.

Duration of the Kundalini process.

The duration of the Kundalini process may take different lengths of time. This depends on the individual path. In the already mentioned Kundalini handbook it is spoken of about 15-20 years. In a few cases this process may take much shorter. My personal process takes already 21 years, but I expect that it comes to an end very soon (maybe this springtime?). Already after the first year I thought it would only be a matter of a few weeks or days, until my process is complete. But again and again I have noticed that more and new energy blockades - even greater energy blockades - dissolved. Accordingly, the receivable resistance of this part of my aura, which is still compressed, seemed to increase. So, what is compacted, is not noticeable. Therefore, it is impossible to recognize the overall duration based on the current process.

Although the Kundalini process has steadily grown in strength or intensity, I sometimes had the feeling that it would take no end. Of course, I knew that there is an end. But over time, more and more and ever greater energy blockades have been resolved. Often I said inwardly, that this is the bright madness and that behind this incredible aura it must be a plethora of energy. Otherwise I couldn't explain this process. And if once this aura is fully unfolded or developed and all blockades are dissolved, then something great must happen.

By the very fact that there is constantly something changing and that there must be an end, a feeling was able to come in me that it goes forward. Even if things didn't always work out so well, as my ego often wished, through this process I always was encouraged to keep going on and not to lose patience. I had to remember over and over again the end result of this process, for not to lose patience in some situations.

Adapting difficulties of the body.

We live in a time in which themes of self-discovery, self-healing, self-realization and self-development are processed intensively. A corollary is, as already mentioned, that we are reinforced faced with different energies (subtle energies, higher dimensional energies, cosmic energies and so on). These energies are unaccustomed for our bodies. Then, if these unfamiliar energies start pouring too much or too fast into our energy body system, there may be certain difficulties in adjusting and adapting of our body. Here we have then to do with symptoms, which cannot be explained, in fact, with the conventional medicine. In this process the Kundalini energy of man, which is a pulsing energy, may be also in a considerable degree at work here. As already mentioned, we are living in a time of increased exposure of energy and of self-development in which this energy will be awoken in man in a strengthened way.

Regardless of the strength of the awakening, the Kundalini energy has the task to flow through all the energy pathways of our energy body system. By its flow and pulsing manner it solves gradually all possible energy blockades and lets the Aura more and more unfold. At the same time this energy harmonizes the aura centers (chakras, which are transmitting and receiving antennas) one after the other, so that the aura will become more and more receptive to higher dimensional energies. So, the Kundalini ensures that internal higher dimensional energies can flow in and can be incorporated in the aura system. This contributes to the overall harmonization of the energy body system and thus to the energy blockade solution at all possible levels. About this way our mind gets clearance. Once all energy blockades are dissolved, then our mind can be connected along the main power canal over the Crown Chakra with the cosmic consciousness, so as to cancel the limits of mind. As a result skill, talents and gifts can grow as we could not imagine in our wildest dreams. **Thus, the Kundalini energy is something like a pioneer for the liberation of our mind.**

Now it may be that the soul of a person feels a great urge for advancing the liberation of the mind. If the mind of this person (ego), however, has refused to work on his liberation, it may now be that the soul abuts that exemption by creating situations that greater amounts of Kundalini energy will be released in the body. If the man has not ensured in advance to prepare his energy body system for this energy, it may be that this Kundalini awakening now causes greater difficulties. It may also be that large amounts of Kundalini could be released, in case that you are strongly drugged, by making exaggerated meditation exercises or even by deliberately making exercises for Kundalini release.

If the energy body system is not prepared for a particular strength of Kundalini release, there may be adapting and adjusting difficulties of our body, that can strongly strain the body: flashes of light, then chills, hearing voices, from on top of the world to in the depths of despair by the one moment to the next, similar symptoms of schizophrenia, and so on. Such people suddenly can be very highly energy charged and can sometimes be very unbearable. It may also be that such people suddenly (for some moments) are mentally deranged and suffer from a relatively large loss of reality. It may also happen that momentarily the vertebrae of the spine are shifting or the organs in the body are shifting, that the Kundalini energy paves its way pop-like or explosively and that the whole body energy system can be messed up. This can go so far that the functions of the body are completely muddled up (death-like conditions) for a short time, which may be associated simultaneously with extracorporeal experiences. By this way man can come to a limit between "death" and life over a certain period. How this process will run, will here be unpredictable. Here trust is then truly necessary in the highest degree.

If such extreme symptoms emerge, it is very important that you do not get into panic and you do not try to do or to let do things too quickly, that could aggravate the situation even more. For such people it is very important that emotional support is provided for them, that great patience is applied to them and that you care about them, but also that them is given the peace (silence, rest) that they need.

For a certain time, I took in charge of a young woman who had withdrawal symptoms of psychotropic drugs as well as a Kundalini crisis. Experience with this woman showed that one couldn't assign in the respective moments, whether such extreme conditions were based on the withdrawal effects or of Kundalini crisis. It should be well known that even with withdrawal symptoms people can come to the limit between life and "death" as it is also possible at a Kundalini crisis.

I speak of phenomena, for which a diagnosis in the classical sense is not always possible or things are at play that are largely unknown in classical medicine. If such phenomena are getting out of hand, there is no silver bullet and no guarantee of anything, no matter at what measures we let us tempt. Whether we treat these symptoms or not, it may end differently (can go either way out).

The use of medication such as psychotropic drugs should be considered as a last resort and in any case carried out with caution here. If possible, friends, acquaintances or family members should take in charge such a person in his usual familiar environment until he has made a recovery. Of course, situationally doctors or therapists can be consulted. However, the path to psychiatry should be considered as a last resort.

Although I pointed out possible extreme cases, who already happened, it should be made clear that these cases are not the rule and that they are among the really few exceptions. But to my finding (due to personal reports) they seem to accumulate nowadays more and more. In general, the Kundalini experiences can be mastered relatively well, they are anyway there to come to liberation of the mind.

It is really amazing that in spite of the above-described extreme conditions (in the cases known to me) <u>no real harm has arisen</u> to the body. That is why it is so helpful to know about the phenomena associated with the Kundalini energy or other Light Body or transformation processes. With this knowledge it can be removed the breeding ground for certain fears. Because with fear, we run slightly risk to do things that could aggravate the situation even more. **While we have normally to do nothing more than to let happen and to endure, it is natural to explore in extreme cases how far we place our lives in God's hands or/and in the hands of doctors and therapists.**

What do we perceive in others?

There are empathic people who perceive, how we feel. Sometimes they perceive it as unpleasant or bad energy. But represents it really our true nature? I do not think so. For as long as we are not aware of our real being, we are showing characters and/or properties that do not correspond to our true nature.

Let us remember that most the time we still feel as a body and not as a spirit. The body is a kind of mask that we play. It got a life of its own, which is on program. We are programmed to do things, that the others love us, that they appreciate us and so on. We are programmed to provide certain services in order to trigger the feeling of recognition both in the other as well as in ourselves. This program prevents us to be as we want really to be.

To get refund the awareness of our divinity, all the effects of these programs have to come to light, so that we can transform them. So if an unpleasant feeling comes in connection with a specific situation (dispute, failure, accident, injury, ...), it will help us best, if we allow this feeling to come, but have in mind that it is only temporary and corresponds not really to our very own essence. So, this feeling can go to give space the feeling of joy and the feeling of love.

So what we perceive in conflict or in uncomfortable situations or what the other persons perceive on us, is only something temporary, unless it does not baffle or faze us. The latter is the case when we have found our true center. Then we cannot really get worked up. Then we would not really more eke out a life on earth (for learning). If

44

we prolong this life anyway, it would be for example for reasons to continue our services to people in the physical form. We could also do it from higher levels. But if it belongs to our soul's plan to be furthermore in physical form for services, we will maintain the physical form, although we would not really need this for ourselves. **Thus, this issue always has something to do with a decision, but not with a necessity.**

So as long as we are still on our spiritual path, we will (unintentionally) show properties that does not correspond to our true nature. Then if anyone thinks he would have a good knowledge of human nature, just because he knows to describe good your characters, characteristics and idiosyncrasies, he deceives himself mightily. So, he takes only something temporary true but not your true nature. **True knowledge of human nature possesses only one who recognizes the Divine in others on the one hand and that the other plays only a role which refers to his own self-image, on the other hand.** A self-image may be incorrect. It is wrong if it is not in conformity with the true self that we are in reality.

When the Buddha had arrived in the state of highest enlightenment, he said first the following, as

Udo Petscher (see: http://www.holofeeling.com/) writes: *"Is not it all completely wonderful!!!??? Is this creation not absolute madness!? I myself and all beings and phenomena which are dreamed by me acquire at the same moment the enlightenment of their lives/existences! "*

If we are not in this state, we are not aware of this. Then we see in us and in others something that just doesn't correspond to our true divine nature. And yet, the true divine nature exists in each of us. Therefore, I think the following is the rightful judgment: We see in others both: his true divinity <u>as well</u> his outwardly projected (selfish) properties, wherein the thing that strikes us about him, always has the function of reflecting my own self-assessment. Only if we bring these two perspectives into a synthesis, we make in my view a legitimate opinion on us and the other and enable us to take steps towards to our enlightenment.

I know that I know nothing and I also know that I know everything. If I would only say: "I know that I know nothing", I would not be able to get to know because I would not be open for the true knowledge. I would always deny it. If I would say on the other side: "I know everything", I would be just as little open to the true knowledge, because I would be indeed close for further knowledge. I would think, I already know everything. Only the "both" brings us to the true knowledge, because all is open and all new ideas are welcome.

For this Udo Petscher continues to write: "... *Under these conditions, the wish to teach my fellow men will be a paradoxical matter. What I want to teach someone if this someone is a part of myself? If I consider myself as a wise man and if I lift me up to a teacher, every part of me must be my teacher. A "normal teacher" who believes to have to teach an ignorant little, thus elevates himself to an ignorant, because his opponent is indeed only a mental projection of his own self. A real teacher realizes that he, strictly speaking, should always be the student of all and therefore also of his own pupils. So, you have to lower yourself to a student of all, if you want to be a really wise teacher! Only if you realize that everything and everyone has been created by God only to be able to grow out of itself/himself, you can really be wise".*

Our all creativity.

Perhaps it should still be noted that we can certainly pursue material goals. With regard to our happiness this does no harm as long as we pursue these goals playfully and thus gather such experiences that we want to gather up. We finally are all creators who always create something and are associated with what we have created. Therefore, we should not even have to find ourselves, because it's not really about self-discovery or perfection. In reality, we are entire, whole and complete. **So, why to search for what we really are?** The point is rather that we are still discovering our creativity again and again and that we seek after deciding what we want to do, we want to be or we want to experience. Only in this sense our creativity makes really fun. But if we believe that the implementation of any tangible goals could make us happier or more fully or whole or complete, we are at a fundamental thinking error that never lets satisfy our longings or aspirations. Such faith keeps us away from the awareness of our true divinity.

Primarily, this book is intended to draw attention to the Kundalini because particularly at the present time it awakens more and more in people. Since we humans are still unconscious creators, the Kundalini can come into our lives, without it is consciously activated in us. Its activation can be initiated spontaneously. Therefore, it is beneficial to know about it, if it enters into our lives in some way. Of course we can also consciously activate this energy and work with it. If you want to activate it in your body, then you should do this only, if you are well prepared for it or if you feel an inner impulse for it or if you has received corresponding characters (signs of heaven). I make this recommendation because this energy is a very powerful energy. Once it enters into our lives, then we can stop it anymore. This should be clear to everyone. Nevertheless, the Kundalini energy is a blessing, because it is relevant to our spiritual development.

Closing remarks.

Perhaps it should still be noted that it is not my intention to provide guidance to get faster to the awareness of our divinity. First and foremost I would like to point out that at any moment we have the choice to do two things. **Either** we can do something that binds us furthermore to the matter and that lets us remain in our unconscious creativity. **Or** we can do something which lifts us energetically up and which leads us to conscious creativity. In the above image, I have tried to represent this principle schematically. But this does not necessarily mean that things that are fun (traveling, driving carousel or otherwise) always hinder this realization. They do it only when you seek your fortune in the outside and when you do not really realize that you carry everything inside you what you need to your true happiness.

Well, for those who have to deal with symptoms associated with the Kundalini energy that cause them great difficulty, I recommend to do, inter alia: They should, of course, primarily try to keep calm. Then it can be very helpful to talk to other people, for example, through appropriate forums. **Try also to inform your partner, neighbor or even your**

doctor, if he is open for it. Sometimes it helps a lot if the other can be there for you and if necessary can also provide for you, if you are just very weak. Of course, every now and then medications can also help to relieve symptoms. Mostly, however, the symptoms disappear after a certain time by itself (without medication). Certainly there is no silver bullet for this. Try therefore, to learn to feel intuitively what is most helpful for the moment for you!

We also live in an age of enlightenment. I spoke of the conventional medicine which still has a need for education in these modern symptoms. **In this respect, I appeal also to the representatives of conventional medicine, to familiarize themselves with the processes of subtle energy body and the so-called Light Body symptoms.** It needs the synergy of all disciplines in the medical and healing system, see my website:

http://www.franzguenter-leicht.info/

Literature and sources.

Holofeeling: www.holofeeling.com

Chakra Handbook; Sharamon, Shalia & Baginski and Bodo J.
http://www.amazon.com/The-Chakra-Handbook-Shalila-Sharamon/dp/094152485X

Kundalini and the Chakras", Genevieve Lewis Paulson
http://www.amazon.com/Kundalini-Chakras-Evolution-Lifetime-Llewellyns/dp/0875425925

The Subtle Body; Cyndi Dale
http://www.amazon.de/The-Subtle-Body-Encyclopedia-Energetic/dp/1591796717

My website
http://www.franzguenter-leicht.info